clinical
effectiveness

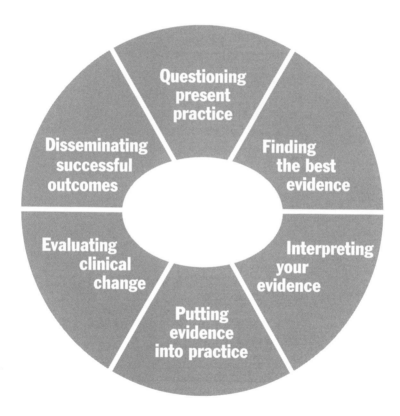

Questioning present practice

Disseminating successful outcomes

Finding the best evidence

Evaluating clinical change

Interpreting your evidence

Putting evidence into practice

a practical guide
for the community nurse

by Cheryll Adams with a foreword by Dr JA Muir Gray

Published by
The Community Practitioners'
& Health Visitors' Association
40 Bermondsey Street
London SE1 3UD
020 7939 7000

first edition October 2000
second edition October 2003
ISBN 1872278 59 0

Written by
Cheryll Adams

Design by
Emphasis Publishing Limited

This work was undertaken by the Community Practitioners' and Health Visitors' Association which originally received funding from the National Institute for Clinical Excellence. The views expressed in this publication are those of the author and not necessarily those of the Institute.

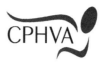

CPHVA

clinical
effectiveness

a practical guide
for the community nurse

2nd edition

Cheryll Adams
MSc, BSc (HONS), DMS, RN, RHV
Professional Officer,
Research and Practice Development
Community Practitioners' and Health Visitors' Association

with a foreword by

Dr JA Muir Gray
CBE, DSc, MD, FRCP (Glasgow & London)
Director, National electronic Library for Health and,
Programme Director, National Screening Committee

Expert reviews on first edition

'This book is a landmark in community nursing and sets the agenda for the 21st Century'

Dr JA Muir Gray,
Director, National electronic Library for Health and
Programme Director, National Screening Committee

'wonderfully easy-to-follow text combining practical procedures or steps with clear explanations of underlying theoretical concepts...one of those books you keep on going back to...puts the implementation process within the reach of all primary care professionals'

Health Service Journal

'well organised progressing logically through the steps of clinical effectiveness'

Nursing Times

'the book has proved to be invaluable to me and has proved to be an excellent learning tool that is clear and easy to understand'

Student Health Visitor, Cheltenham and Tewkesbury

'a must for the community nurse's bookshelf'

Nurse Practitioner

Featured 'Document of the Week'

National electronic Library for Health

Contents

Acknowledgements

Many people made the first edition of this book possible. Most importantly my family and colleagues at the CPHVA in particular Toni Turner, then editior of the *Community Practitioner* who commissioned the original articles and suggested they should result in a book.

The Department of Health and the National Institute for Clinical Excellence were then supporting the work of the CPHVA clinical effectiveness department as part of their core audit programme. This book and my work was in part, a product of that funding although the views expressed are my own and not those of the funding bodies.

My thanks must also go to Professor Martin Severs, Director of the Institute of Medicine, Health and Social Care in Portsmouth. He was a tremendous support and enthusiast when I first entered the world of 'Clinical Effectiveness'. Thanks also to my past research and health visiting colleagues in Portsmouth who have helped me to explore the challenges of integrating research with practice and in so doing making it accessible to the practitioner.

Valuable assistance with the preparation of this second edition has been given by Indi Munasinghe, Information Resources Officer at the CPHVA, Melanie Danforth, Editor of the Community Practioner Journal and Dr Neil Brocklehurst, Senior Lecturer at City University, London.

Cheryll Adams, October 2003

Preface to 2nd edition

This book, which is based on a series of articles published in the *Community Practitioner* journal, will introduce all community nurses to the processes involved in clinical effectiveness. From an understanding of these processes you can start to question the evidence-base for your practice and if necessary make changes to improve its quality and thus its effectiveness. The book also discusses ways of sharing outcomes so that others may learn from them, saving time and benefiting patient care. The book is designed so it can be read as a whole or individual chapters selected to inform particular activities.

The author has welcomed the positive feedback on the first edition from members of many different professional groups suggesting that the book has proved useful in supporting the development of their understanding of the clinical effectiveness agenda. In the short time since it was published, UK health departments have put in place a variety of mechanisms to support practitioners in responding to the quality agenda. At field level however, the greatest challenge often remains having the time to stand back and reflect on existing practice.

Whilst the essential content remains unchanged, this second edition has been revised and updated and describes new resources which are accessible to most health visitors and community nurses with the greatly improved provision of information technology (IT) in their workplaces.

Cheryll Adams, October 2003

Foreword to 1st edition (October 2000)

The community nurse on the north Norfolk coast has always been one of the paradigm users of the National electronic Library for Health. She might also be a paradigm user for this book. Spending most of her time in a car, on the road, calling in occasionally at a health centre or community services office, the community nurse has had to lead a life far away from the library or librarian. When she has time in the evening, in many places the library is locked and the librarian unavailable; some community nurses have until recently had no access at all to a library; although one hopes this situation no longer exists the fact of life is that library services for community practitioners have always been scanty at best.

Thus the community nurse has always had to be self-reliant and had to manage the knowledge she needs to survive in her lonely job. Community nurses have also been supportive of one another in exchanging knowledge and know-how in the course of their work.

This book recognises the role that knowledge management has in community nursing and identifies ways in which skills can be improved and developed. It describes how the organisations in which community nurses work have to change to be more supportive to the individual practitioner.

The nurse on the north Norfolk coast will, however, in the near future be able to access the world wide web in any house she visits, for the web will be on television and every house will have access. The job for the community nurse will then change again, but not too much. Nurses have for a long time seen themselves as facilitators who enable the decisions made by patients and not people who hoard knowledge and use the power knowledge can bring. Again this book identifies the contribution that the individual practitioner makes to clinical practice in the age of the internet.

This book is a landmark book in community nursing and sets the agenda for the 21st century.

JA Muir Gray CBE DSc MD FRCP (Glasgow & London)
Director, National electronic Library for Health and.
Programme Director, National Screening Committee

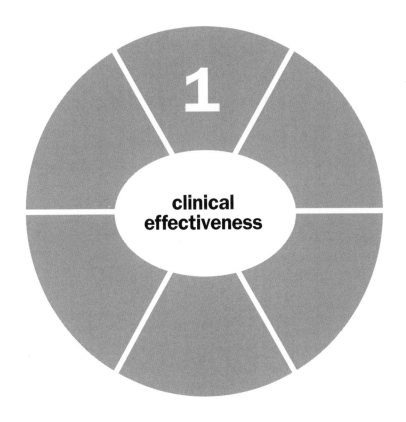

1

clinical
effectiveness

1
Questioning present practice

To be clinically effective involves primarily ensuring that your practice is based on the best available evidence of effectiveness and meets your clients' requirements. Furthermore, that you implement any change to practice within a framework of review and evaluation. Once you have achieved clinically effective practice it is important to share your experience with others so that they may also benefit from it.

Testing your knowledge

Could you explain these terms?
(Answers at the end of this chapter)
1   Clinical effectiveness
2   Clinical governance
3   Evidence-based practice
4   Critical appraisal
5   Cochrane collaboration
6   Systematic review
7   Randomised controlled trial
8   Meta-analysis
9   Clinical audit
10   Health outcomes

The Department of Health White Paper, *A First Class Service* 1998,[1] proposed a framework for ensuring that the NHS provides a quality service. It suggested a 10-year plan with the aim of ensuring that there is 'fair access to prompt high quality care wherever a patient is treated in the NHS'. It is the task of the clinicians to ensure that the care which they are providing is as efficient and clinically effective as possible within the current boundaries of knowledge. This personal responsibility is a key part of the clinical governance agenda.

In order to achieve clinical effectiveness it is necessary to determine best practice, to apply it in day-to-day practice and to make sure that it works (Figure 1).[2] For many community nurses this is a new way of working and there are new skills to

Figure 1: The process required to achieve clinical effectiveness

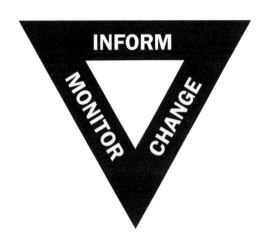

be acquired before they can be expected to respond to the challenges this new culture brings. The CPHVA has produced a number of publications to facilitate this process.[3-6] This book is designed to complement them.

Questioning present practice

In order to respond to the clinical effectiveness agenda, nurses must start questioning their routine practice. What is its evidence-base? Could it be performed more effectively?

An analogy to gardening can demonstrate the value of practising in this way. A gardener plants out some seedlings. In time she notices that some are twice the size of others. An ordinary gardener may not question why this should be. A 'gardening-effectiveness' gardener will question why some plants have grown larger. Has she unintentionally given them more fertiliser? Are they receiving more light or water? At this point her husband opens the window and throws out the water he has been using to wash the vegetables. It lands on the taller seedlings. Her question has been answered! They are getting more water.

As with the 'gardening-effectiveness' gardener in health care we must now start to question continuously our practice and ask which interventions achieve real health gain for our clients.

Stage 1: Choosing an aspect of practice

There are a number of stages to ensuring that your practice is clinically effective. First, you must chose a specific aspect of care or service delivery which you want to examine or question.

An example could be maternal diet and breastfeeding. We know that maternal diet is important but you might question how important it actually is to successful breastfeeding. We never quantify its importance. If a good diet is essential how can a health visitor or midwife most effectively ensure the quality of a breastfeeding mother's diet when that mother is living in poverty? These days many mothers are very conscious of what constitutes good nutrition and they eat appropriately. What community nurses need to be able to determine is when they need to suggest nutritional improvement. What is the cut-off point between a good and a bad diet? What is the value of vitamin supplements and so on? Furthermore, how can they intervene most effectively? Which strategies for improving nutrition in their clients work?

As can be seen from this example the fairly simple questions – how important is maternal diet to breastfeeding and when and how should health visitors and midwives suggest nutritional improvement – would in fact require a great deal of time to answer. Nevertheless, they could lead to a more targeted, evidence-based approach to offering nutritional advice to breastfeeding mothers.

Stage 2: Finding the right question

As a busy practitioner it is essential that a question is asked that can be answered in a realistic amount of time. Questions therefore need to be specific. Normally they are generated by practice and as such may be able to be answered by the nurse herself or another nurse. It is always worth asking colleagues whether they can answer your question before you embark on time-consuming literature searches. If they can offer an answer you should ask them to back it with good evidence. If they can't then you can plan a search of the literature and other sources of information.

Stage 3: Framing a question

In order to undertake a literature search it is essential that the question be very focused otherwise it will be impossible to deal with the quantity of information found.

Chambers and Booth[7] suggest that there should be a number of aspects to a clinical question.

It should be:

○ simple
○ specific
○ realistic
○ important
○ capable of being answered
○ agreed and owned by those who will be involved in any changes resulting
○ implementable
○ about a topic where change will be possible.

The above is a useful check list to consider your question against. In framing a specific question you need to consider four aspects to the question. These are: the patient or problem; the intervention; the setting, and the outcome.

For example, faced with concerns regarding a high level of teenage pregnancies in a local secondary school there would be a desire to come up with an effective intervention to reduce teenage pregnancies in the school. You could ask: 'Can issuing free condoms in secondary schools reduce the number of teenage pregnancies?' (see box overleaf for four aspects).

Examples of other specific questions might be: 'Can the

The four aspects are met as follows:

○ the patient or problem would be the number
  of teenage pregnancies
○ the intervention would be the issue of condoms
○ the setting would be the school
○ the outcome would be a reduction in the number
  of teenage pregnancies.

Edinburgh Postnatal Depression Scale be used by community nurses during routine contacts other than in the postnatal period to detect depression in their clients?'; 'Is brief health education for smoking cessation delivered during one-to-one contacts by practice nurses effective in improving health behaviour?'; 'Could reflexology be used by district nurses to help control pain in terminally ill patients being treated at home?' Can you determine the four aspects of each question?

Sometimes a general question has its place and must be answered before a more specific question can be generated. You could ask: 'How can school nurses influence teenage pregnancy rates in secondary schools?' This is a much less specific question and will not provide specific answers. What it will provide though is a general overview of possible interventions. These can then be considered and those realistic for the circumstance looked at in more detail with a specific question (this will be discussed in more depth in chapter 2).

How to set up a local clinical effectiveness group with interested colleagues

There are many advantages to working with colleagues when questioning the evidence-base of your professional practice. Setting up a clinical effectiveness group can have a number of advantages, both professional and personal:

○ group support for the development of evidence-based
  practice

○ several heads are better than one!
○ professional development
○ a more rigorous outcome
○ development of skills in critical thinking
○ improved communication
○ to promote an awareness of research
○ to support the provision of optimal care for your patients
○ to give credibility to outcomes suggested for implementation.

Research has shown[8] that successful groups include the following features:

○ support from management
○ lunch-time meetings with refreshments
○ the participants have undergone critical appraisal skills training.

A suggested way forward is to:

○ obtain management backing
○ identify interested staff; six to eight is the maximum size for useful discussion. The group could be uni or multi-professional depending on the proposed agenda
○ arrange critical appraisal skills training for these staff
○ arrange a first meeting
○ let the group decide the format of their meetings; ie frequency, venue, content
○ identify a link to your management group
○ elect a chair/facilitator (rotate regularly)
○ decide the terms of reference for the group
○ consider how you will evaluate the group.

While clinical effectiveness groups have a similar format to journal clubs where members bring papers they have found for discussion, they generally differ in that the approach is much more focused. Papers are selected to answer a specific question and then critically appraised. The outcome of the appraisals is discussed in relation to their value for informing or changing practice. Nevertheless, there is always advantage in appraising current papers brought by members which appear to be relevant to your practice. Without undertaking a literature search, however, you may not be aware of other relevant papers which offer conflicting outcomes to papers which have caught your eye.

A suggested format for examining practice in the group[8,9]

Meeting one, stage 1
Consider a key clinical/professional problem (points to consider are cost, frequency and priority of the problem) and then formulate a specific question about it which requires answering.

Stage 2
One member searches for evidence to answer the question. The librarian in your local postgraduate medical library should be able to help; many offer training in searching the research databases, some will do the searching for you and provide print-outs of relevant research papers. Most professional bodies can also provide search facilities for their members. If you have access to the internet you can use the National electronic Library for Health (NeLH) (www.nelh.nhs.uk) site to search all the main health databases yourself.

Meeting two, stage 3
Members decide which research papers are most relevant, the papers are ordered and distributed to members to appraise critically, (critical appraisal is covered in chapter 3 of this book).

Meeting three, stage 4
The chosen papers and results of the critical appraisal are discussed in terms of their quality and relevance to practice. Brief details of the outcomes are recorded. These could be circulated to colleagues.

Stage 5

If appropriate the management team is made aware of any recommendations from the discussion in a briefing paper.

In some instances no research will be found and a suggestion might be sent to the local research and development (R&D) department that this is an area of need. Alternatively a group member or colleague might be interested in undertaking relevant research perhaps as part of other academic studies. In the short term though any recommendations will have to be reached on the basis of expert opinion and professional consensus. Rather than relying on the views of just the group members, other information might be sought from relevant national bodies working in that area.

The group's format will evolve with its membership. Until the members feel confident in searching for robust research themselves, much value can be gained from appraising existing systematic reviews relevant to your professional practice. The best source being the Cochrane database (see chapter 2).

A number of other useful sources of evidence reviews are 'Clinical Evidence' published by the British Medical Journal (www.clinicalevidence.com) also the 'Evidence briefings' published by the Health Development Agency (www.hda-online.org.uk/evidence) and the NHS Centre for Reviews and Dissemination Effectiveness Bulletins (www.york.ac.uk/inst/crd). This chapter introduced readers to the first step in clinical effectiveness – questioning present practice. The next chapter will discuss how to find the best research evidence to answer your question.

Further information

Further useful information on the processes of clinical effectiveness can be found in the NHS publication, Achieving Effective Practice[10], which can be located on the internet: http://www.doh.gov.uk/pub/docs/doh.aep.pdf

Definitions of terms

Clinical effectiveness is the extent to which specific interventions when deployed in the field for a particular patient or population do what they intend to do ie, maintain and improve health and secure the greatest possible health gain from the available resources.[2]

Clinical governance is a framework through which the NHS organisations are accountable for continuously improving the quality of their services and safeguarding high standards of care by creating an environment in which excellence in clinical care will flourish[1]

Evidence-based practice is the conscientious, explicit and judicious use of current best evidence in making decisions about the care of individual patients. The practice of evidence-based health care means integrating individual clinical expertise with the best available external, clinical evidence from systematic research.[11]

Critical appraisal is the process whereby research (qualitative or quantitative) is assessed to determine its validity and suitability for informing practice.

The Cochrane Collaboration is an international initiative in which people from many different countries produce and keep up-to-date systematic reviews of research from randomised controlled trials of all forms of health care. The results of these reviews are stored on the Cochrane database making them accessible to health practitioners and decision makers.

Systematic review is a review or summary of the literature in which evidence on a topic has been systematically identified, appraised and summarised according to pre-determined criteria.

Randomised controlled trial is a research technique where the subjects are randomly assigned to either an intervention or a control group. In this way it is intended that the characteristics of the two groups will be similar. The two groups are compared at the end of the trial to see whether the intervention has led to differences.

Meta-analysis is a statistical technique whereby the results of several randomised controlled trials can be summarised.

Clinical audit is a quality improvement process that seeks to improve patient care and outcomes through systematic review of care against explicit quality criteria and the implementation of change. Aspects of the structure, processes, and outcomes of care are selected and systematically evaluated against explicit criteria. Where indicated, changes are implemented at an individual, team or service level and further monitoring is used to confirm improvement in healthcare delivery.[12]

Health outcomes are the effects of a particular intervention or series of interventions on the health of a client or client group. They can refer to effects on individuals, communities and whole populations. Measures of health outcome have three important characteristics: an intervention is needed; the outcome must be attributable to the intervention; and the outcome is a change in health status or health gain.

References

1   NHS Executive. A first class service. Leeds: NHS Executive, 1998.

2   NHS Executive. Promoting clinical effectiveness. Leeds: NHS Executive, 1996.

3   Hudson R. Demonstrating effectiveness: compiling the evidence. *Health Visitor* 1997; 70: 12, 459-461.

4   Hudson R. Clinical effectiveness: a practical approach. *Nursing in General Practice* 1997; 3, 4-5.

5   Community Practitioners' and Health Visitors' Association. Clinical effectiveness information pack. London: CPHVA, 1998.

6   Adams C, Forester S. Clinical Governance in Primary Care and Public Health Practice. London: CPHVA, 2002.

7   Chambers R, Boath E. Clinical effectiveness and Clinical Governance made easy. Oxford: Radcliffe Medical Press, 2nd ed 2001.

8   Bandolier 1997; No 43, 7.

9   Sackett D *et al.* Evidence-based medicine: how to practice and teach EBM. London: Churchill Livingstone, 2nd ed 2000.

10   NHS Executive. Achieving effective practice – a clinical effectiveness and research information pack for nurses, midwives and health visitors. Leeds: NHS Executive, 1998. Web only: www.doh.gov.uk/pub/docs/doh.aep.pdf

11   Sackett DL *et al.* 'Evidence-based medicine: what it is and what it isn't' (editorial). *British Medical Journal* 1996; 312, 7023: 71-72.

12   National Institute for Clinical Excellence. Principles for Best Practice in Clinical Audit. Oxford: Radcliffe Medical Press 2002.

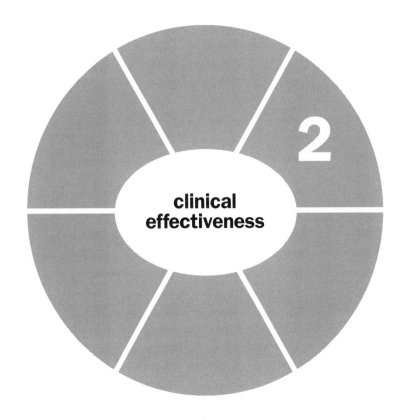

clinical
effectiveness

2

2
Finding the best evidence

As with most activities, success in finding best evidence comes with practice. Providing the opportunities for practice is a management as well as a professional issue. As the clinical governance agenda is implemented the need for every community nurse to gain the skills to question their practice and underpin it with best evidence has increased in relevance. So also has their need to access computers and computer training.

Sources of information and best evidence

Community nurses can and do use a huge number of sources of information, but which are most reliable? The most accessible source of information is usually colleagues; it may also be a very efficient source but how do you know? You know if colleagues make suggestions which work. Professional experience should never be under-rated. Just because no-one has conducted research to examine an area of practice it doesn't mean that there isn't good evidence based on professional experience available which is worthy of consideration. It is often necessary, however, to also look to the literature for published research to inform your practice.

When wanting to obtain evidence from the literature where do you start? In 1995 Chalmers and Altman reported that every year over 20,000 biomedical journals are published which include two million health-related papers.[1] These numbers are constantly growing with new journals being published every year. Furthermore there are thousands of related books. Books are not generally considered to be the best source of research evidence because of the time delay in publishing and the fact that the information they offer may quickly become dated. Nevertheless they remain a useful source of wider discussion around a topic area.

There are two good general sources of scientific and medical evidence available to practitioners – libraries and the internet via the worldwide web. Another good source may be specialist associations or indeed specialists. Although not every community nurse has good access to library services in their workplaces increasing numbers have access to the internet. Furthermore, access to training to use IT facilities is proliferating.

Access to information resources and the research literature

There is no better time to be asking your Primary Care Trust/Organisation to facilitate your access to research evidence. Indeed the Department of Health has supported the provision of such information with improved internet access for all staff and access to the NHSnet and the National electronic Library for Health. This latter is an information 'super-highway' for all staff working in the health service. The aim is that these resources will improve the efficiency, effectiveness and equity of health-care delivery by offering all NHS staff access to up-to-date research via the major medical and nursing databases. Eventually they should be available in every NHS workplace through computer terminals.[2] Already they are available in general practitioners' surgeries and increasingly in the nurses' and health visitors' offices.

Even if you have trouble accessing libraries, the NHSnet or the internet an arrangement for literature searches to be performed on your behalf should be possible with the local health care, postgraduate medical or university library. Where libraries are many miles from a nurse's base it may be possible to ask management to provide satellite information points in a local centre. Access to the internet and main medical databases could be provided at these points. They could also be visited regularly by the librarian to provide training for searching the databases. This service would ensure that every member of staff has access to the research literature even if they do not have the time or skills to find relevant articles themselves.

Many specialist databases are now accessible free of charge via the web. Also, there is provision for accessing articles in full text through international data archiving services.

Which evidence sources are most useful?

But where can you find the best evidence quickly? Fortunately there are a number of sources of appraised research and these are always the best starting place.

Of particular value is the Cochrane database of systematic reviews. This is now available free of charge through NHSnet and the NeLH. An Athens login and password are required to access the full text of reviews and instructions for arranging this are on the NeLH site. A systematic review is a review or summary of the literature in which evidence on a topic has been systematically identified, appraised and summarised according to pre-determined criteria. The reviewer includes not only the published but also, where available, unpublished literature. If you can find a systematic review which answers your practice question then this will be very helpful and save a great deal of time.

Another excellent source of systematically reviewed and appraised research is *Clinical Evidence* which is available as a book and via the NeLH. Published by the BMJ publishing group, publishers of the *British Medical Journal* (BMJ) it provides best research evidence on the effects of common clinical interventions. Much of its content is of interest and relevance to community nurses, particularly practice and district nurses and should underpin their practice. The web version is searchable. (For further details 020 7383 6270 or www.clinicalevidence.org) The BMJ also has a very useful free searchable database on the net which will yield research and other discussion articles on most areas of health care. It is one of the most visited health sites (www.bmj.com)

Also very helpful are the effectiveness bulletins produced by the York Centre for Reviews and Dissemination (CRD).

These systematic reviews address a variety of topics of interest to community nurses including:

- ○ preventing unintentional injuries in children and young adults
- ○ mental health promotion in high risk groups
- ○ preventing and reducing the adverse effects of unintended teenage pregnancies
- ○ management of head lice
- ○ pre-school hearing, and speech, language and vision screening
- ○ the prevention and treatment of pressure sores
- ○ preventing falls and subsequent injuries in older people
- ○ promoting the initiation of breastfeeding
- ○ the prevention and treatment of obesity
- ○ preventing the uptake of smoking in young people
- ○ compression therapy for venous leg ulcers.
- ○ homeopathy
- ○ acupuncture
- ○ interventions for the treatment and management of CFS/ME.

Copies are obtainable from CRD (01904 434565). The abstracts are short and well presented.

Another good source is *Bandolier* (www.jr2.ox.ac.uk/ Bandolier), which publishes commentaries on research and attempts to make the understanding of research outcomes more accessible to the general clinician. Published monthly this is essentially targeted at doctors but has many items of general interest. Another useful source of appraised research may be journals of secondary research. *Evidence-based Nursing* and its sister journals, *Evidence-based Medicine, Evidence-based Mental Health* and *Evidence-based Paediatrics* offer research reviews. They publish selected original and review articles that are chosen for their quality and ability to inform practice. Each article is accompanied by an expert commentary.

The internet is proving a colossal source of information on

any topic. Unfortunately though much material being entered onto the web is not peer-reviewed so it must be used with extreme caution. The best site for evaluated websites relevant to nursing practice is NMAP (http://nmap.ac.uk) To evaluate a website you need to consider the following:

○ the credibility of the author
○ how up to date the site is
○ the relevance of the information to the topic
○ whether information is referenced and the credibility of the reference sources
○ whether the site includes contact details for the author and to obtain further information.

Also helpful are the National Research Register (NRR) and the Research Findings Register (ReFeR) which are available via the NeLH. These provide a fairly comprehensive picture of research which is currently taking place in the NHS. If you can't find any published information to support your topic area it may be helpful to know whether there is research taking place so that you can contact the researchers for details.

Table 1 summarises the type of information available from the most useful electronic databases of research and audit.

Table 1: Electronic databases

Cochrane Library (www.cochrane.org)
The Cochrane Library was set up to provide systematic reviews of research on important areas of health care. It initially focused on maternity services but now covers most areas of health care. The bias is medical. Furthermore it tends to discuss treatment options rather than service delivery but nevertheless it is an invaluable source of information and should be your starting point. The database is actually three databases: the Cochrane Database of Systematic Reviews (CDSR), the Cochrane Controlled Trials Register (CCTR) and the Database of Abstracts of Reviews of Effectiveness (DARE). All the material included in Cochrane has been quality screened.

TRIP (www.ceres.uwcm.ac.uk/frameset.cfm?section=trip)
This is a meta-catalogue of evidence-based healthcare resources which are available on the internet.

CINAHL (www.cinahl.com)
This large database covers details of articles related to nursing, health education and the allied professions. Being American it has a somewhat North American bias. The contents are not quality assessed.

British Nursing Index (BNI) (www.bniplus.co.uk/)
This is a British index of nursing articles and is very useful, although the contents are not peer reviewed and there are no abstracts available.

Medline (www.ncbi.nlm.nih.gov/PubMed/)
This is the computerised version of Index Medicus. It is very useful, containing a vast amount of information. It has details of articles from over 3700 biomedical journals. Its weaknesses for nurses are the medical and North American bias. It is not quality assessed.

HealthPromis (healthpromis.hda-online.org.uk)
Bibliographic database published by the Health Development Agency (HDA). Identifies the evidence of what works to improve people's health and reduce inequalities.

National Research Register (www.doh.gov.uk/research/nrr.htm)
Database of NHS research in progress.

PsychoInfo
This contains details of articles on all aspects of psychiatry and psychology. It is not quality assessed.

National Research Register (www.doh.gov.uk/research/nrr.html)
Database of NHS research in progress.

National electronic Library for Health (www.nelh.nhs.uk)
By far the best one stop source for health information giving direct access to all of the most useful, high quality research and practice databases.

NMAP (nmap.ac.uk)
The UK's free academic gateway to high qualtiy internet resources in nursing, midwifery, health visiting and the allied health professions.

Searching the electronic databases

We have established that there are many potential sources of information that might be used to inform your practice. What we must now consider is how to search these sources efficiently. Obviously in some circumstances it may be most practical to arrange for a library search. This is quick and efficient for the practitioner but the search will only be as good as the information provided to the searcher. The librarian must make decisions in your absence and in so doing may lose information which you would have chosen to keep.

Chapter 1 discussed the need to have a specific question to answer. This becomes very apparent when you start to search the literature. Without a specific question you will retrieve an unmanageable quantity of information. Furthermore, it is essential to use the right terminology or key words. For example, literature on postnatal depression is more likely to be found on Medline using the term postpartum depression. A librarian can help you to choose your key words and there is a published thesaurus of medical terms to aid the clinician wanting to conduct a search on Medline, using so-called MeSH terms. Their structure resembles that of a tree. Major headings are those such as depression and asthma and these branch into narrower subject terms. If you use a term which is not a MeSH term you are offered a choice of words with similar meanings. You then decide which to use.

The next step is to decide how you will search in order to filter the information you are looking for from all the available information. If, for example, you are searching for information on enuresis you may want to limit your search to enuresis in pre-school children, to a particular area such as management, to robust research studies such as randomised controlled trials (see chapter 1) and to English language papers. In this way you sift out a great deal of information and you end up with a more focused and manageable outcome. There are options given on the screen to help you narrow your search.

For the community nurse new to searching the literature this may seem the most confusing step. Published search strategies and guidance are available to help you.[3-6] The search strategy is adapted to support your personal needs. You can search by looking for your search terms in the title, abstract, main body or for the author's name in papers. Once again booking a session with a librarian will be invaluable in helping you get started.

Example of a search strategy in response to the question:

What is the best treatment for head lice?
   Using these terms should elicit a good cross section of
      published materials:

   "head lice and treat*" and "effective* or standard* or
      guideline* or good practice*"

   NB 'and', 'or' and 'not' are words which help to refine the
   search. * or $ (CINAHL and Medline) are known as the
   'Wild Cards' and allow you to search for truncated words.
   In this case these might include 'treatment, treatments,
   effectiveness etc'.

To save time it is best to start your search with the most robust
and most relevant sources of information. The Cochrane databases are always a good start and can be entered via the
NeLH which also offers a large number of alternative databases to search. Cochrane may have limited content relevant
to some community nursing needs but it is quick to search and
includes the most robust research evidence available. You may
then choose a nursing or medical database. For a psychiatric
topic such as postnatal depression PsychoInfo may prove most
useful. For enuresis it could be CINAHL, British Nursing Index
or Medline. For peripheral vascular disease in diabetes
Medline should yield up to date research. There can be considerable overlap in the contents of the different databases.
   Your search will provide you with a list of available literature on your chosen subject. It may be titles and authors or
abstracts. Abstracts are most useful as they offer an insight into
the focus of the paper. The list can then be compared to your
practice question and the papers which appear to be most relevant obtained. It is important when choosing literature to be
aware of not only that which appears to answer your question

Table 2: Hierarchy of research evidence[7]

○ Strong evidence from at least one systematic review of multiple well-designed randomised controlled trials.

○ Strong evidence from at least one properly designed randomised controlled trial of an appropriate size.

○ Evidence from well-designed trials without randomisation, single group pre-post, cohort, time series or matched case-controlled studies.

○ Evidence from well-designed non-experimental studies from more than one centre or research group.

○ Opinions of respected authorities, based on clinical evidence, descriptive studies or reports of expert committees.

but also of that which is based on good quality research. There is a hierarchy of quality in research (Table 2). Answers provided by systematic reviews are thought to be considerably more reliable than those of a respected authority as they combine the results of a number of pieces of research. Many areas of research are not covered by systematic reviews in particular qualitative research. In this instance look out for other reviews which may not be as thorough but are helpful in providing an overview of your area of interest.

Other useful sources of evidence

Professional bodies may be able to provide literature searches, copies of published papers and loan books. The CPHVA provides internet training days. There are also many specialist organisations which offer information services to practitioners. Due to their specialist interests they are usually aware of the latest research as soon as it is published. Examples are the National Childbirth Trust (0870 444 8707), the National Asthma Campaign (020 7226 2260) and the Enuresis Resource and Information Centre – ERIC (0117 960 3060). A very useful service is that provided by the Midwives Information and Resource Service (MIDIRS). Although this is most relevant to midwives there is a great deal of overlap with health visiting. For a small fee a detailed search, with abstracts, is available (0800 581009). There is also an internet search facility (www.midirs.org) The organisation publishes a list of available topics with over 70 concerning aspects of postnatal care. Through the NeLH you can access vast amounts of other useful clinical information such as SIGN and NICE guidelines, care pathways, information on alternative therapies and much more.

Using the evidence

Putting evidence into practice is the subject of chapter 4. First though the outcome of your search must be considered in relation to the area of practice you are questioning. This is most useful if done with colleagues; for example, in a clinical effectiveness group as discussed in chapter 1. In some instances it may be useful to contact the authors of research for further details. Their contact details are usually published with the paper. Your decisions will also be much more valid if you have applied a critical appraisal process to your chosen papers. Critical appraisal will be considered in chapter 3, and offers a system for quality screening of research before applying it to practice. Having reached a conclusion to your search it is useful to record the process you have gone through to discuss and share with colleagues and managers. Figure 1 gives a summary of the whole process for conducting a literature search.

This chapter has considered where and how to access

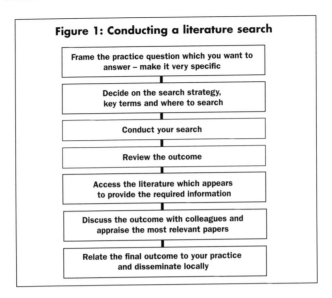

Figure 1: Conducting a literature search

Frame the practice question which you want to answer – make it very specific

Decide on the search strategy, key terms and where to search

Conduct your search

Review the outcome

Access the literature which appears to provide the required information

Discuss the outcome with colleagues and appraise the most relevant papers

Relate the final outcome to your practice and disseminate locally

sound evidence of effective practice. It has also described the principles of conducting a literature search using electronic databases. Success in developing this skill will be dependent on opportunities to practice.

References

1   Chalmers I, Altman D. Systematic reviews. London: BMJ Publishing Group, 1995.

2   NHS Executive. Information for health 1998. Leeds: NHS Executive, 1998.

3   Greenhalgh T. How to read a paper. London: BMJ Publishing Group, 2nd edition, 2000.

4   Chambers R, Boath E. Clinical effectiveness and clinical governance made easy. Oxford: Radcliffe Medical Press, 2nd edition 2001.

5   Muir Gray JA. Evidence-based health care: how to make health policy and management decisions. London: Churchill Livingstone, 2nd edition, 2001.

6   Sackett D et al. Evidence-based medicine: how to practice and teach EBM. London: Churchill Livingstone, 2nd edition, 2000.

7   Bandolier 1995; 12.1.

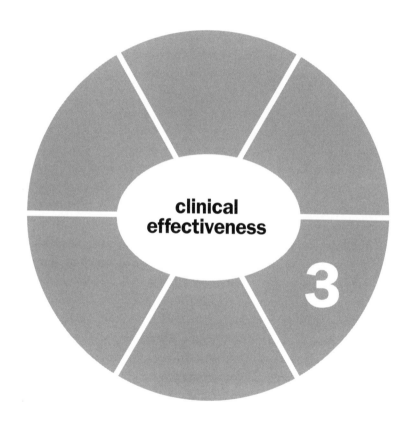

clinical
effectiveness

3

3
Interpreting your evidence

This chapter suggests simple ways of quality-assuring the information you have found.

This process is called 'critical appraisal'. Essentially critical appraisal is about looking objectively at evidence and determining what it means, whether it is robust and whether it is relevant to your practice.

Background

Before embarking on a discussion of the processes of critical appraisal it may be helpful to understand why this process has become so important, indeed why the evidence-based practice culture is receiving such prominence.

Evidence-based medicine has been described by Sackett et al,[1] one of the main proponents of the culture, as being the 'conscientious, explicit and judicious use of current best evidence in making decisions about the care of individual patients'. Over the past 20 years there has been increasing recognition that many health care decisions are based on tradition rather than evidence. Indeed lives have been lost when the results of research have taken many years to be implemented.[2]

In his foreword to the White Paper A First Class Service[3] the then Secretary of State for Health stated: 'Clinical decisions should be based on the best possible evidence of effectiveness, and all staff should be up-to-date with the latest developments in the field.' In order to be able to use the best evidence we must therefore have mechanisms for finding and determining what is the best evidence. Hence the requirement of health professionals to gain skills and understanding in assessing the quality and relevance of research. The results of robust research can then be combined in systematic reviews (secondary research), to inform guideline production and to be disseminated to health professionals.

Sources of evidence

We have seen previously there are two sources of evidence, primary and secondary. Primary sources are often of unknown quality and may be based on subjective or objective interpretation of information. That is, they may be merely a description of what the author has seen and thinks was happening or they may be based on a more systematic and objective collection of information. Either way, vast quantities of primary research are published every year and can prove a real challenge to the inexperienced researcher who is required to interpret them for their relevance.

Secondary sources of evidence are becoming increasingly available and are of much more value to the practitioner who wishes to question the evidence underpinning his or her practice but has neither the time nor skills to embark on a lengthy exercise. Secondary sources have done part of the work for you. As we have seen previously the best secondary sources are systematic reviews. Unlike traditional reviews these accumulate evidence in a systematic way, quality-assure the collected data and make recommendations based on the outcome of the review. A good systematic review will publish its methodology in full. Professional life would be made easy if we could rely on the results of systematic reviews and merely apply them in practice. The reality is that the focus of the review is not necessarily exactly the same as that of the practitioner. Furthermore, the review may contain a number of biases related to its purpose or methodology and we must be alert to these. They will be discussed in more depth below.

Another concept to grasp before looking critically at evidence is whether the evidence is based on quantitative or qualitative research. Your approach to appraising each will be slightly different as it will be for secondary sources. Quantitative research measures fact and usually employs statistics to compute and describe the results. Qualitative research, on the other hand, explores the reasons behind the observations, introducing a more 'human' element. I often think of quantitative research as providing the bones to understanding some aspect of health care – if a treatment works, for example – while qualitative research puts the flesh on the bones – what a patient's views of the treatment are. We have known for many years that smoking lowers life expectancy – this was as a result of quantitative research. Knowing how to reduce the incidence of smoking, however, requires qualitative research to determine, among other things, the human factors which affect an individual's decision to smoke. Only then can services be targeted at reducing the incidence of smoking and its long-term effects on health. The flesh is a much more complex mechanism than is the skeleton.

Qualitative research has in the past tended to attract a poor press from the medical profession, which is often concerned with making black-and-white decisions on behalf of its patients. For example, which drug or treatment will be effective is a question answered by a quantitative methodology. Another use for quantitative research would be for understanding the epidemiology of certain conditions. The fact that we know cardiovascular disease is often related to a history of smoking, obesity and lack of exercise was determined from huge (quantitative) population studies.

It is becoming increasingly popular to back quantitative research with qualitative research. An important quantitative study of interventions for postnatal depression by Appleby et al[4] concluded that although the quantitative research suggested that medication was as, or more, effective than counselling for treating postnatal depression, women would, if given the choice, in general opt for counselling. Since the patient should always be the focus for our choice of health care this qualitative aspect to the research was very important.

The problem with any research is that it will only be as sound as the methodology employed. Good research will also identify and try to eliminate bias. Bias should be accounted for in the results and discussed in the research report conclusions.

Armed with an understanding of the broad categories which research falls into, we can now consider how it may be quality-assured. How do you start? There are a number of quality filters you can apply to your evidence. They are not foolproof in sorting out good evidence from less good, but they will help the less experienced or busy practitioner. They are particularly useful when you are trying to choose papers from the results of a library search.

Primary filters

1 Is the evidence relevant to your practice question?
If it isn't look elsewhere.

2 Was the research based on a systematic review?
The process of systematic review both filters for quality and combines the findings of robust research but systematic reviews are usually only applied to quantitative research.

3 Has the research been chosen for inclusion in a secondary source of research?
Research entered onto the Cochrane databases or published in *Clinical Evidence*[5] has undergone an intensive quality screen first. Furthermore, it will be accompanied by details of why it was chosen which is very helpful to the non-expert in appraisal. This also applies to journals providing secondary sources of research such as *Evidence-Based Nursing*. It must be remembered though that this filter is unlikely to have been applied to qualitative research.

4 Where was the article published?
Was it in a serious scientific journal targeting researchers and educationists as well as clinicians, or in a journal more targeted to clinicians? You expect to find articles in scientific journals arising from research. These are written in a specific style with

an abstract summarising the research, followed by an introduction, methods, results, discussion and conclusion. The evidence they offer is usually of a higher scientific quality than that of articles in many general professional journals which are often descriptive in style.

5 Was the evidence peer reviewed before being published?
If peer review is a pre-requisite of publication the journal should state this. Peer review requires the article to be commented on by one or two independent subject experts before a decision is made to publish. If it has been peer reviewed then it has gone through the journal's quality screen prior to publication.

Obviously these filters cannot alone determine the quality of the evidence but if it has passed them then you can presume there is a better likelihood of it being of a superior quality to evidence that has not. This particularly applies to questions 2 and 3. You quickly learn which journals publish secondary or peer reviewed research, so it can guide your choice of evidence for further attention.

The difficulty comes with many areas of health care where large research studies employing good research methodology do not exist. The evidence you may find is practice experience recorded in nursing journals in a descriptive format. It may be very valid but this can be more difficult to prove. This chapter will focus on how to critically appraise research making it through the primary filters. As you develop the skills of critical appraisal you should find they will also start to influence your interpretation of all evidence.

Appraising research

Essentially there are three questions to ask of any evidence[6]
  ○ can you trust it? (reliability)
  ○ what does it mean? (outcomes)
  ○ is it relevant to your practice? (relevance).

In order to answer these questions it is necessary to examine how the research was done, the results and the interpretation of the results. On first exposure evidence can sound very convincing. Every practitioner will benefit from understanding the skills for considering it more critically.

Where do you start?
There are some excellent check-lists available which support the process of critical appraisal.[7-11] You should be guided by these but we will discuss the important issues you need to consider when appraising both qualitative and quantitative research. Systematic reviews will be considered separately.

Relevance
The title may offer some clue as to whether the evidence is relevant to your requirements, though titles can be misleading. The abstract, if available, may be more helpful. It outlines how the research was done, the results obtained and the conclusions drawn. What you must determine is whether the results are generalisable to other populations, in particular the one which you are studying. To give an example: the research may have considered what influences the smoking habits of teenage girls, using a university student population as the subject group. You are interested in how you can influence the incidence of smoking in teenage mothers. Are these two groups of teenagers the same? I would suggest that their attitudes could be very different. While the research might offer useful information it may not be relevant to your needs and it would be prudent to look for other sources more relevant to your target group.

Reliability and outcomes
The reliability of any evidence is often its weakness. It should be possible to replicate most research based on the methodology reported if it is reliable. When you read research it should have:
- ○ a clear aim (purpose)
- ○ methodology which is appropriate for achieving the aim

○ opportunities for bias should have been considered and eliminated as far as possible
○ the results and any statistics should be clearly reported
○ conclusions drawn should be based on the results and original aims.

Aim

This should have been arrived at from studying previous published work and finding a gap in knowledge. The author should record how it was determined by describing that work. It should be clearly stated and reflected in the other sections of the study.

Methodology

This is key to the value of the study. The type of methodology chosen should be the most appropriate to meet the aim of the study. It should be as robust as possible. A randomised controlled trial is the 'gold' standard of quantitative research. This is where subjects are randomly assigned to a control or experimental group. Providing the total numbers are large enough it has the advantage of producing two groups which should be closely matched for personal and clinical characteristics. If this methodology has not been possible but the authors have attempted to match the experimental group with a control group based on certain features, the results will be more believable than if they have not. In the case of qualitative research a control group may not be employed but the sample group should be as representative as possible of the population being studied. All research will have benefited considerably too, if it has been piloted prior to the main study.

The sample size in a quantitative research study is key to the reliability of the results. Different methodologies require different sample sizes but the larger the sample the greater the reliability of the results. Sample sizes are determined statistically by what is known as a power calculation, and this should be described in the methods section. The researcher aims to keep as many as possible of the original sample group in the study until the end. If there has been a large drop out rate then the results will be less valid. Good quantitative research will calculate the results on what is known as an 'intention to treat' basis, including the number who have dropped out. This dilutes the result but a positive result becomes even more powerful. When appraising all research it is important to look at the sample size, how it is justified and how the results were calculated or derived from the data collected.

Furthermore, the population studied should be representative of the population required to answer the research question. You need to ask who was excluded and why?

Bias

When reading the methodology it is important to be alert to any source of bias. We have already mentioned some, such as not having a representative sample, nor an appropriate sample size, nor allowing for the drop out in the calculations. Other sources of bias can be related to whether the same person measured the outcomes or conducted the interviews. Furthermore, whether the outcomes were measured based on standardised tests or human interpretation. When outcomes are assessed blind in quantitative research it is much more powerful. This means that the assessor is unaware of the status of the subject in the study he/she is testing. Assessing blind helps to remove human bias.

Other sources of bias could occur during a study. The study might be running a large child safety campaign and wanting to look at attendances at the accident and emergency (A&E) department before and after the campaign. If, coincidentally, the television ran a series of programmes on preventing childhood accidents, it should concede that any reduction in attendances at A&E might have been biased by the television programmes. The presence of the television programmes is what is known as a 'confounding factor'.

Results

These should be clear and simple and comprehensible to the non-researcher. In particular any statistics should have an explanation. Response rates should be reported. Numbers should add up. You must query the validity of any evidence based on research where the response rate is low unless a satisfactory explanation is given and it has been adjusted for in the calculations.

Conclusions

These must reflect the aims and the results. No new information should occur in the conclusion. Have alternative explanations been considered for the outcomes? Are the conclusions justified? You must consider if the sample size is small or there has been a large drop out, whether it is reasonable to conclude a definitive answer. Most importantly the conclusions should make clear recommendations for practice if justified from the study. You must decide whether these recommendations could be reasonably applied in your practice.

A final point to consider is whether there is any conflict of interest. Who sponsored the research, for example?

The perfect research study involving human subjects is virtually impossible to achieve. Academics also rarely agree in full on how results should be interpreted so don't be daunted. One of the most useful ways of gaining practice in critical appraisal is with other colleagues in a group.

Appraising systematic reviews

These are likely to be a type of research which you will want to consider. As you will recall a systematic review collects, appraises and summarises research in response to a particular practice question.

There are three additional important questions to ask.
○ How were the papers identified?
○ How was the quality of the papers assessed?
○ How were the results summarised?

Identification of papers

A good systematic review will look for evidence from the published and unpublished literature and will use a variety of different sources to cross-check that as much evidence as possible has been collected. In order to do this it must address a clearly defined question and there should be clearly defined criteria of what will be included. In some instances the amount of evidence initially uncovered will be very large. If the question is not clearly focused then it will be impossible to reduce the evidence to a manageable size. A discussion of how questions should be framed was included in chapter 1.

Quality assessment

The review methodology must have a system for determining the quality and strength of evidence of the papers. This system should be reported in the methods section and have required the agreement of at least two researchers. There are a number of published systems.[12,13]

Summary of results

The results should be presented clearly in table form to allow the reader to judge whether the interpretation was valid. The table should provide necessary details about the studies such as sample size, age range and length of follow-up. Many systematic reviews include a meta-analysis which combines similar results in a summary which is a more powerful result as it includes a larger number of participants. The reader must decide whether it was reasonable to combine the studies which were combined.

Table 1 explains common statistics used in systematic reviews. Figure 1 illustrates how the results may be produced.

Table 1: Statistics often reported in systematic review articles

Odds ratio This is one measure of clinical effectiveness. If the odds ratio is equal to one then the effect of the intervention is no different from no intervention. If the odds ratio is more or less than one then the effect is smaller or greater than no intervention.

Risk ratio The risk ratio is similar to the odds ratio but it measures the ratio between proportions.

Numbers needed to treat This is the number of people who need to receive an intervention for one successful outcome.

Confidence interval The confidence interval gives a measure of the precision (or uncertainty) of study results for making generalisations about the population of all such patients. A 95 per cent confidence interval is the range of values within which we can be 95 per cent sure that the population value lies. If the confidence interval is from less than one to more than one the results are less significant as indeed they are if the confidence interval is wide. The greater the number of subjects in a study the narrower the confidence interval (the greater the confidence).

Meta-analysis This combines the results of several randomised controlled trials to give a more powerful result.

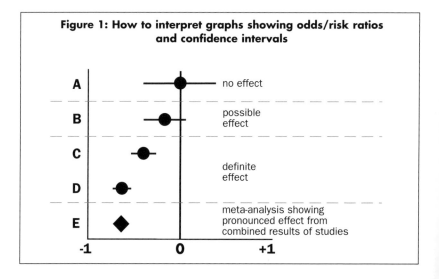

Figure 1: How to interpret graphs showing odds/risk ratios and confidence intervals

A — no effect

B — possible effect

C — definite effect

D

E — meta-analysis showing pronounced effect from combined results of studies

-1   0   +1

Conclusion

For those readers who are keen to further their knowledge in this area I would recommend that you investigate the possibility of undertaking a course on critical appraisal or evidence-based practice. Courses are run by many local research and development departments and university departments and also by the UK wide Primary Care Research Networks which can be joined by community nurses. For details of your local Network www.ukf-pcrn.org/ or Tel: 01623 486 635. Other sources of courses are the Critical Appraisal Skills Programme in Oxford (CASP – 01865 226968 or www.phru.org.uk/~casp/), Centres for Evidence-based Child Health in London (020 7905 2606) and Scotland (0131 225 7324) and the Centre for Evidence-based Health Care in Oxford (01865 286942/286941). Also available are distance learning materials produced by the CASP unit. Alternatively there are a number of useful publications available which cover this subject.[7-13]

A large number of concepts have been discussed in this chapter. Having some understanding of them will sharpen your ability to look critically at evidence before considering using it in practice. The next chapter will focus on how to change practice by incorporating new evidence.

References

1 Sackett D *et al*. Evidence-based medicine: what it is and what it isn't (editorial). *British Medical Journal* 1996; 312, 7023: 71-72.

2 Chalmers I, Altman D. Systematic reviews. London: BMJ Publishing, 1995.

3 NHS Executive. A first class service. Leeds: NHS Executive, 1998.

4 Appleby L, Warner R, Whitton A, Faragher B. A controlled study of fluoxetine and cognitive-behavioural counselling in the treatment of postnatal depression. *British Medical Journal* 1997; 314, 932-936.

5 BMJ Publishing Group. Clinical Evidence. London: BMJ Publishing Group, 2003. www.clinicalevidence.co.uk.

6 NHS Executive. Achieving effective practice. Leeds: NHS Executive, 1998. Web only: www.doh.gov.uk/nhsexec/aep.htm

7 Critical Appraisal Skills Programme. Evidence-based health care. Open learning resources. Anglia and Oxford: NHS Executive, 1999.

8 Crombie I. The pocket guide to critical appraisal. London: BMJ Publishing, 1998.

9 Sackett D, Richardson W, Rosenberg, Haynes R. Evidence-based medicine – how to practice and teach EBM. London: Churchill Livingstone, 2nd edition, 2000.

10 Greenhalgh T. How to read a paper. The basis of evidence based medicine. London: BMJ Publishing, 2nd edition, 2000.

11 Gray JAM. Evidence-based healthcare: how to make health policy and management decisions. London: Churchill Livingstone, 2nd edition, 2001.

12 Chambers R. Boath E. Clinical effectiveness and clinical governance made easy. Oxford: Radcliffe Medical Press, 2nd edition, 2000.

13 Abbott P, Sapsford R. Research methods for nurses and the caring professions. Buckingham: Open University Press, 2nd edition, 1998.

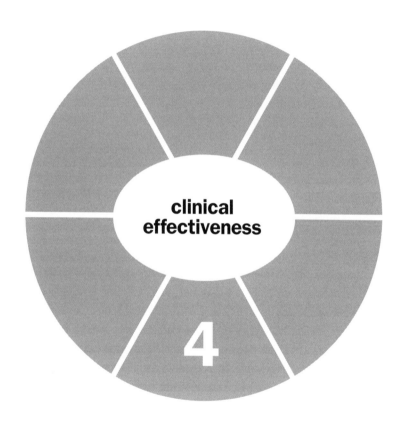

clinical
effectiveness

4

4
Putting evidence into practice

Opportunities and skills for finding the best evidence to inform practice have increased dramatically over the past few years. Successfully changing practice to incorporate new evidence, however, remains a considerable challenge. It is a challenge community nurses must take up in line with the clinical governance agenda to improve the quality of health care.[1] This chapter offers a practical focus and insight to this key area in the clinical effectiveness cycle.

Managing change components are now added to many courses, both professional and management, indicating the need for all staff to gain skills in this area. Knowing how to change practice is, however, only the start. The reality of applying theory to practice can prove difficult as it is dependent on several factors. The change process is also extremely complex. First, you need to consider your own professional practice:

○ Where and when did you get the information which you gave to your last patient?

○ When did you learn any skill you have used recently?

○ What influences you to change practice or incorporate new information into your existing practice?

○ When you have made a successful change in your practice what made it successful?

In many instances you will still be using information or skills which you picked up when you trained. When you learn a skill for the first time, in the author's experience, you often remember it and it influences your practice for many years. If you consider something as simple as brushing your teeth, when the dental hygienist suggests a new technique it can be difficult to make the change from the one you are familiar with. I believe that our practice is heavily influenced by inspiring teachers who provide us with skills or information for the first time. Certainly, I could still list the lecturers who have been most influential on my practice.

To make a change then, the change agent (a person or situation) must be influential in order to persuade us to make the change. This could be a colleague or local or government policy. Change in practice, as we have seen, should be based on sound evidence. Every health professional has a responsibility to respond to guidance from the National Institute for Clinical Excellence (NICE) and the National Service Frameworks – use of such guidance will be monitored by the Commission for Health Improvement. This could be a powerful force for change.

Consider changes that you have made successfully, either in your own life or professionally. What were the main influences on you which led to you making the change? Making any change usually requires a considerable personal effort and is only achieved when the forces to change are greater than the forces not to change.[2] Some of these forces are particularly powerful. Consider seat belt legislation. Seat belts were fitted to cars long before it was mandatory to wear them. Although the public were well aware of the evidence that they saved lives this was not a strong enough influence for many individuals to use their seat belts. It was only by making the wearing of seat belts mandatory that the influence (the threat of conviction) was powerful enough to ensure that most drivers started to use them.

We are all subject to such influences. Consider the influences that would be felt by a health visitor if, in response to the research evidence, she or he tried to discontinue routine weighing of babies in a clinic. You will now be starting to understand the multitude of different forces which can influence the process of change. Logically, in order to make a change successfully, it is helpful to first consider the nature of such forces.

Theoretical models for change

It is useful to understand the theory behind the change process. It explains the behaviour of health professionals and underpins strategies for change and is well summarised in the *Effective Health Care Bulletin* on 'Getting evidence into practice',[3] which is available free to all interested health care professionals by telephoning 020 7290 2928 or on the web: www.york.ac.uk/inst/crd

Influences on change

Taking the useful management mnemonic, 'PESTEL', we can start to examine the factors which can influence the change we wish to make:
- ○ Political
- ○ Environmental
- ○ Sociocultural
- ○ Technological
- ○ Economic
- ○ Legal.

If we briefly apply these areas to the need to change practice in the light of new evidence, we will start to see the broader factors that influence the process. These are outlined below.

Political
There is a powerful political drive to make our practice more evidence-based. Indeed it is government policy, as set out in *The NHS Plan*[4] and in *A First Class Service*[5] and *Making a Difference.*[1]

Environmental
Environmental factors, such as the availability of a suitable infrastructure and access to education and communication systems, must be present to support the change process.

Sociocultural
There are often powerful sociocultural factors such as public and professional beliefs and attitudes which delay the acceptance of new research. Equally there may be powerful social reasons for acceptance, such as unacceptable levels of mortality or morbidity.

Technological
Technology can facilitate or delay the process; for example, by access to equipment and information systems.

Economic

This can be a very important influence. While some evidence will improve the quality of the service for patients it may also increase costs, reducing the availability of other services. Furthermore, additional training or staff may be required incurring still further costs.

Legal

There may be legal considerations such as the safety of new treatments and whether staff are adequately trained to apply them.

Barriers to change: fieldworkers' perspective – a needs assessment

I would like to share the results of two workshops I ran looking at the challenges of the clinical effectiveness agenda. The participants, all community nurses, were asked what they felt the greatest problems and barriers would be in their practice to proposed changes outlined in a number of fictitious scenarios. The scenarios involved setting up evidence-based services for managing postnatal depression, childhood asthma and preventing accidents in the elderly. Participants' responses, shown in Table 1, make interesting reading. Table 2 highlights proposed solutions suggested by the same nurses. Other research into barriers to nurse utilisation of research highlights lack of time and resources as the main barriers.[6]

Table 1: Problems in introducing change

Problems anticipated

○ A fragmented service.*

○ Conflicts between professional views.

○ No specific standards.

○ A lack of epidemiological data.

○ A lack of resources.

○ Having a universal understanding of the issues.

* It may be significant that this was mentioned by most of the groups.

Barriers to effective change

○ Stigmas associated with the condition (postnatal depression).
○ Too time-intensive.
○ Social perceptions.
○ Overlap of services.
○ Lack of research into effective strategies.
○ Difficulties in team working.
○ No national strategy.

Table 2: Suggested solutions

○ More joint training.
○ Raise public awareness of the conditions.
○ Routine screening.
○ More proactive working by the community nurses.
○ Improved IT.
○ Nurses should determine priorities, not government.
○ More large research studies to inform practice.
○ Better evaluation.
○ Shifts in resources.
○ Consumer satisfaction surveys.
○ A national lead.
○ Evidence-based guidelines.

National perspective – research-based

A number of national projects have attempted to find solutions to the challenge of moving research into practice. Indeed the government has commissioned a systematic review on this subject[3] also on managing organisational change.[7] Other projects include GRiPP (Getting Research into Purchasing and Practice), STEP (South Thames Evidence-Based Practice Project), ACE (the Assisting Clinical Effectiveness programme) and FACTS (the Framework for Appropriate Care Throughout Sheffield).[7,8]

Particularly well known is the PACE (Promoting Action on Clinical Effectiveness) project led by the King's Fund in

London.[9,10] This set out to understand how change can be implemented in clinical practice. It involved introducing change in 16 different sites in England and monitoring the process. The outcome showed that introducing change 'is a costly and messy business, but that it can be achieved if there is sound evidence on which to base the work and if a project management approach is adopted. It is not a logical process and it takes a lot of time, people and materials to drive the work on'.[10]

The review from the NHS Centre for Reviews and Dissemination at York was based on 44 systematic reviews. It concluded:[3]

○ it is essential that there are routine mechanisms by which individual and organisational change can occur
○ as well as individual beliefs, attitudes and knowledge, other factors including the organisational, economic and community environments of the practitioner are also important
○ any attempt to bring about change should first involve a 'diagnostic analysis' to identify factors likely to influence the proposed change. Choice of dissemination and implementation interventions should be guided by the analysis and informed by knowledge of relevant research
○ a range of interventions has been shown to be effective in changing professional behaviour in some circumstances. Multi-faceted interventions targeting different barriers to change are more likely to be effective than single interventions
○ successful strategies to change practice need to be adequately resourced and require people with appropriate knowledge and skills
○ any systematic approach to changing professional practice should include plans to monitor and evaluate, and to maintain and reinforce any change.

We now know some of the theory behind successfully incorporating research findings into practice and the essential features for planning a change in practice. We have also seen that achieving practice change may be complex and require many factors in order to be successful.

Change in practice

As a busy community nurse it is important not to be put off by these complexities but rather to involve as many of the stakeholders in the planning as possible. You could act as a facilitator rather than attempt to manage the process yourself. I would suggest there are a number of stages to the process. Let's consider these in relation to a proposed change for managing head lice in the community.

Over the past few years wet-combing has become the treatment of choice for managing head lice in the community. Its popularity has grown because of concerns about the use of the available pharmacological preparations, which are insecticides.

You are aware of a local epidemic of head lice and wet-combing has not kept it in check. You pose the question: 'What is the most effective intervention for managing head lice in childhood?' Your search yields a number of pieces of secondary research; studies which have critically appraised research literature.[11-15] They have considered three possible interventions: wet-combing, insecticide-based pharmacological products, and herbal and aromatherapy treatments. Combing has not been properly evaluated, and neither have the herbal/aromatherapy treatments. The suggestion is that combing could be effective but success is related to the frequency of the combing and the skill of the operator. It is useful, however, for confirming the presence of live lice. The only intervention with evidence of effectiveness is the use of insecticides.

Discussing these findings with colleagues and your manager you decide that it is necessary to change the advice that you are giving to parents for the management of head lice. While you could simply change your personal advice this would lead to confusion. It is essential that every health professional advising on the management of head lice gives the same advice. Let's presume you are a health visitor or school nurse and are given management support to become involved in implementing the research findings across your health Trust/Organisation.

Stage one

Stage one is to consider who the stakeholders would be in making such a change and involve them. There are many but the main ones are parents, your local public health department, practice nurses, health visitors, school nurses, community nurse managers, schools, general practitioners and pharmacists. The stakeholder with the main responsibility and the broadest overview is the public health department.

Stage two

Stage two is to liaise with your director of public health and the other stakeholders and share your concerns and desire to see a prompt change in local policy based on the latest research. This public health department should be aware of the problem and the research and may already be working on a new policy for head lice management. If not you must make a good case for suggesting the change.

Stage three

Once a local policy has been agreed it is necessary to consider an implementation plan and who will lead the implementation process. While community nurses may not currently be involved in this process, they could be, in line with policy on public health. Certainly at the primary care level the primary health care team of nurses and general practitioners need to be working together to implement the policy. Indeed those nurses who are nurse prescribers are now qualified to prescribe some pharmaceutical insecticides for the management of head lice. It would be useful for each practice to plan an audit of the effectiveness of the current policies in managing head lice in the practice.

Stage four

It can be useful to perform a SWOT analysis. This is a management tool which allows you to consider the strengths, weaknesses, opportunities and threats involved in making a particular change. In this instance these might be:

Strengths
- ○ The change will be based on best current research outcomes.
- ○ The change will be applied to the whole district.
- ○ The change will be led by credible health professionals from public health, community nursing and general practice.

Weaknesses
- ○ Lack of knowledge of the true scale of the problem.
- ○ A lack of public and professional acceptance of the use of insecticides.
- ○ Inadequate links between local educational providers and practice needs.
- ○ Cross-professional communication may be poor.
- ○ If your district is large the community services may be fragmented.

Opportunities
- ○ The change should bring about a significant reduction in head lice infestation.
- ○ Equity of management of head lice in your district/health authority.
- ○ Public education on head lice management.
- ○ To improve contact tracing.
- ○ To involve all the stakeholders.
- ○ To help improve cross-professional communication.

Threats
- ○ Public disquiet about the use of insecticides.
- ○ The cost of additional prescribing of pharmacological products.

○ Professional attitudes to the management of head lice.
○ Availability of resources to support the plan.

Stage five

Based on the results of the SWOT analysis a plan can then be drawn up for implementing the change. The production of a local standard or policy by the public health department for the management of head lice should encourage equity in local management. Furthermore, it allows for an audit to be conducted to review progress.

Before introducing change it is also important to both discuss it with and listen to feedback from the stakeholders involved. This will identify any possible problems in advance. It may be interesting at this point to revisit the potential barriers to change highlighted by field staff and listed in Table 1. The plan should consider:

○ the reasons for the change
○ the policy or guideline (evidence-based)
○ how the policy will be disseminated
○ the possible impact on clinical staff
○ the educational needs of staff
○ a campaign to educate the public
○ the requirements for contact tracing
○ how the change will be monitored and evaluated
○ a time-scale for full implementation.

Essential to successful change will be effective communication. All staff involved should be fully informed of the plan. They are more likely to co-operate with it if they can see an incentive for themselves or their patients. While the management of head lice is considered a necessity for community staff it is also a source of frustration as epidemics are so common and the public do not always understand, or co-operate with, their role in the management of the epidemic. A planned campaign to tackle head lice using the best available evidence for effective management and involving professionals and the public should be an incentive for staff co-operation.

When you start to consider the needs of a public education campaign you can begin to see why achieving successful change can be time-consuming and expensive. Professionals may be persuaded to change their practice by local policies and research evidence. The public may be harder to persuade in this instance. There is little value in changing the policy for the management of head lice if the public will not comply with the new one. Achieving public co-operation may be the real challenge. Such has been the strength of media reports condemning the use of insecticides and promoting wet-combing that it will be hard to change this culture. Imaginative techniques will be needed to alter current thinking. Lessons could no doubt be learned from commercial companies whose marketing departments are very skilled at altering public beliefs.

A useful summary of techniques for changing professional practice is included in part seven of the NHSE publication, *Achieving Effective Practice*.[16] See also the *Effective Health Care Bulletin*, 'Getting evidence into practice'.[3] These techniques include:

○ providing feedback on current practice
○ education
○ standard-setting, involving practitioners
○ provision of clinical guidelines from a credible source
○ using opinion leaders (local experts) to propagate credible information
○ use of quality improvement tools
○ using a marketing strategy and techniques
○ imposing legislation on aspects of clinical practice
○ the provision of reminders.

Techniques for changing public opinion include:

○ good communication
○ use of the media
○ offering incentives (for example, improved health)
○ dissemination of robust evidence

○ use of local change leaders (for example, community nurses).

In fact the NHS systematic review[12] for the management of head lice was published in June 1999 and disseminated to senior managers. Have its findings been implemented in your health district yet? If not you might inquire why not? An article in the Community Practitioner Journal in 2000 describes how one health organisation took a community approach to reducing head lice infection[17]. I have used it as an example for managing change by community nurses. In reality, currently one might expect the process to be led by the public health department, with whom community nurses might or might not collaborate. Nevertheless it is the primary care staff who have direct access to the public and they can contribute useful local information to the implementation plan if they are given the opportunity. This opportunity should come in line with public health policy.[18]

Key principles for success

We have considered the challenge of moving research evidence into everyday practice from the health professional's point of view and that of the user, local practice and the health service. From these discussions it is possible to draw out some key principles which underpin success. These are summarised in Table 3. They are:

○ be sure of what you want to achieve and its relevance to practice and the health of the local population
○ gain management support for making the change
○ gain the support of the stakeholders
○ ask the professionals to identify what they anticipate will be the local barriers to change and how they feel they may be overcome
○ perform a PESTEL and a SWOT analysis

○ make a clear plan which includes specific interventions for the public and professionals. Furthermore the plan should be realistic and relevant to the local situation
○ communicate your plan to the stakeholders
○ recruit a credible change leader
○ chose a method or methods for making the change which is/are suitable to the conditions
○ build in evaluation and opportunities for audit
○ if making a district-wide change, conduct a pilot before introducing the change across the whole area. This will highlight difficulties that can be rectified at an early stage
○ having achieved successful change tell other people how you did it.

These principles can be applied at the Trust or local level and should help to ensure local ownership of the change. Remember, though, that most change takes time, requires a multi-disciplinary approach and will require real commitment and enthusiasm from those involved.

Table 3: The principle steps of successful change management
○ Plan change
○ Communicate with the stakeholders
○ Make the change
○ Evaluate
○ Disseminate.

Conclusion

While leading a change process is an unfamiliar process for many health professionals those readers who have participated in community development work will be familiar with many of the challenges and processes we have discussed. The government has recognised that community nurses are in a key position to lead change which will benefit the health of their clients.

It is therefore essential that if we are to take up this challenge we learn to initiate, facilitate, participate in or lead change, not just at the practice level but on behalf of much larger client groups. The NHSE document, *A First Class Service*,[5] sets out the government's plans for achieving equity in health care and community nurses have an important part to play.

Further reading

This list is by no means comprehensive but summarises some of the literature which the author has found to be particularly useful.

Evidence-based Health Care. Unit 4, Critical Appraisal Skills Programme. Open Learning Resources. NHS Executive, 2nd edition, 2002.
This offers a very useful distance learning approach to the subject. The workbook contains a great deal of very helpful information.

Getting Evidence into Practice. NHS Centre for Reviews and Dissemination. Effective Health Care Bulletin. 1999; 5.1.
This summarises the research evidence for managing the process for incorporating research into practice.

Evidence-based Health Care. Muir Gray JA. Churchill Livingstone, 2nd edition, 2001.[7]
This book contains many items of interest and value to anyone wanting to explore the whole issue of evidence-based health care in more depth.

Experience, Evidence and Everyday Practice, Dunning M, Abi-Aad, Gilbert D, Hutton H, Brown C. London: King's Fund Publishing, 1999.[10]
This reports on the outcomes from the PACE project, and as such, is an extremely useful book for anyone undertaking clinical governance work.

Achieving Effective Practice. NHS Executive, 1998.[16]
This exceptionally useful publication contains 10 papers discussing different aspects of clinical effectiveness. It is now only available on the web.

Organisational Change. Iles V, Sutherland K. NCCSDO, 2001.[6]
This incredibly useful book reviews models for change and the evidence surrounding them. Available free: 020 7612 7980 or email: sdo@lshtm.ac.uk

References

1 Department of Health. Making a difference: strengthening the nursing, midwifery and health visiting contribution to health and healthcare. London: The Stationery Office, 1999.

2 Lewin K. Field theory in social science. London: Harper, 1951.

3 NHS Centre for Reviews and Dissemination. Getting evidence into practice. *Effective Health Care Bulletin* 5, 1; 1999.

4 NHS Executive. The NHS Plan. Leeds: NHS Executive, 2000.

5 NHS Executive. A first class service. Leeds: NHS Executive, 1998.

6 Griffiths J et al. Barriers to research implementation by community nurses. *British Journal of Community Nursing* 2001; 6, 10: 501-510.

7 Iles V, Sutherland K. Organisational change. London: NCCSDO, 2001.

8 Muir Gray J. Evidence-based healthcare. London: Churchill Livingstone, 2nd edition 2001.

9 Mulhall A. Changing practice: the theory. *Nursing Times Clinical Monographs* 1999; 2.

10 Dunning M et al. Turning evidence into everyday practice. London: King's Fund Publishing, 1998.

11 Dunning M et al. Experience, evidence and everyday practice. London: King's Fund Publishing, 1999.

12 NHS Centre for Reviews and Dissemination. Treating head lice and scabies. *Effectiveness Matters*; 4,1; 1999.

13 Dawes M et al. Treatment for head lice. *British Medical Journal* 1999; 318: 385-386.

14 Dodd CS. Interventions for treating head lice. *Database of abstracts of systematic reviews*. The Cochrane Library. Cochrane Collaboration 2003, Issue 1. Oxford: Update Software.

15 BMJ Clinical Evidence. London: BMJ Publishing Group.

16 NHS Executive. Achieving effective practice. Leeds: NHS Executive, 1998. Web only: www.doh.gov.uk/pub/docs/soh.aep.pdf

17 Fee J, Briault V, Long J. A community approach to reducing head lice infection *Community Practitioner* 2000; 73.2: 477-480.

18 Department of Health. Liberating the talents. London: The Stationery Office, 2002.

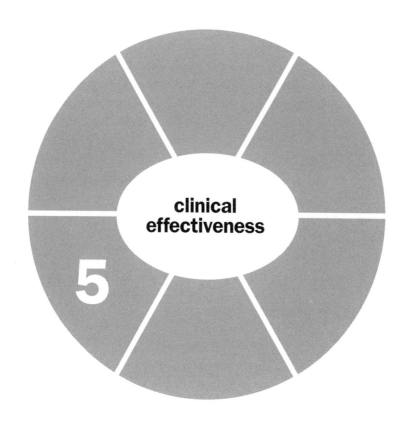

clinical
effectiveness

5

5
Evaluating clinical change

The earlier chapters have shown how community nurses can question the evidence underpinning their practice and take on the clinical effectiveness agenda. One of the most important parts of this agenda is knowing how to quality-assure or evaluate changes in our practice. We must examine whether our objectives or standards are being met and whether the desired outcomes are being achieved for our clients.

The change in practice might relate to the way you plan or deliver your input to the client, or indeed to what you deliver. We are constantly altering our practice in the light of changing circumstances, new evidence of effectiveness or patient requirements. How often, though, do we evaluate these changes? How often do we determine whether it is change for the better?

It is now increasingly important that all health professionals become familiar with the methodologies required for determining the quality of their practice. It is also an essential part of the clinical governance framework.[1] Clinical audit or evaluation should be built into any planned change in practice. Indeed most readers will already have participated in clinical audit or evaluation.

Clinical audit and evaluation

But what is evaluation? You may think you know but actually the term is often loosely used and confused with clinical audit (see Box 1 for definitions). Both processes question whether you have done what you set out to do, but clinical audit examines activity against a standard, guideline or objectives, while evaluation examines it more broadly using similar qualitative or quantitative processes to research. Most clinical audit concerns itself with structure and process, asking whether the activity has met the standard or objectives set for it. It is possible, though, also to audit outcomes. A good evaluation will focus on outcome as much as process and may include clinical audit.

Box 1: Definitions

Clinical audit

Clinical audit is a clinically-led initiative which seeks to improve the quality and outcome of patient care through structured peer review whereby clinicians examine their practices and results against agreed explicit standards and modify their practice where indicated.[2]

Evaluation

Evaluation is the process of making a detailed assessment about what has been achieved and how it has been achieved. It means looking critically at an activity or project to identify what is good about it, what is bad, and what could be improved.[3] It therefore involves an explicit element of judgement, which can incorporate audit measurements.

Research

Research describes activities that involve the planned, systematic collection and/or analysis of data to answer a specific question or to test a precise hypothesis.[4]

Quantitative methods of evaluation often focus on outcomes and qualitative methods are used to look at the processes of care. Qualitative methodologies though may discover outcomes and often provide information relating to why and how outcomes are achieved.

Research and evaluation

A major difference between research and evaluation is that research is designed to produce new knowledge and for the results to be generalisable whereas evaluation results are intended to be of value to the local service. Evaluation looks at a particular area of practice with a specific client group who have not been selected to be a representative sample. The results of an evaluation may therefore not be of value outside the context of that evaluation due to the size and characteristics of the population studied. It is important to understand these differences so as to understand the limitations of a project and commit realistic resources to it.

Assessing quality

To give an example we can consider looking at the effectiveness of running postnatal health promotion groups.

Clinical audit
Clinical audit might examine whether the group is meeting its service objectives in terms of quality. For example:
○ that the group has been made available to every local mother/father with a first child under six months of age
○ that a programme of health education is provided
○ that the timing and content of the group meets the clients' needs.

Methodology might be a client questionnaire to the group's members and a postal questionnaire to a sample of families qualifying for group attendance.

Evaluation
Evaluation, on the other hand, might also examine the group's ability to meet certain outcomes:
○ to improve the parents' social networks
○ to reduce the incidence of postnatal depression
○ to have raised the self-esteem, confidence and knowledge of those attending.

It would utilise methodologies such as a focus group, a before-and-after study using a client questionnaire, a self-esteem scale and a scale for determining the mother's mood such as the Edinburgh Postnatal Depression Scale. It is questioning whether these outcomes have been achieved by comparing the results when the parents first attended the group with results after attending for a agreed period of time. It would also have to take notice of other factors which might have contributed to any improvement in the parent's mental health, as well as examine the process of how the groups were run. The results of the evaluation would be of value locally due to the unique characteristics of the particular group being evaluated. However, they could suggest the need for a more formal research study to determine whether such a service development could be applied elsewhere.

Research
Research would focus on a question such as: 'Can postnatal health promotion groups improve holistic health in first-time mothers and their children?'

In order to answer this question effectively and for the results to be of value to others interested in running such groups the methodology would have to be robust and would normally include a comparison to parents not attending groups. Furthermore, the methodology must be clear about the characteristics of individual groups involved, their members and the sample selection.

Clinical audit
It is estimated the NHS carries out over 20,000 audits a year. Many community nurses may not have appreciated the value of clinical audit as a tool for ensuring quality. It is often confused with managerial audit and hence seen as a process for checking up on them rather than being for quality improvement. It is well recognised that health professionals can generate the most successful clinical audits. Furthermore, a successful audit leads not only to improved quality but also to improved staff morale, staff development and better collaborative working.

Dixon listed common themes from a review of good practice in clinical audit:[4]

○ clinicians, not their managers must choose the subject and aims of the audit. They must focus on elements of the service which they consider to be important
○ the goals of the audit must be explicit
○ the clinicians must be directly involved in data collection
○ the results of the audit must be addressed by managers and commissioners.

Figure 1 highlights the stages of a typical audit and the particular requirements of each stage.

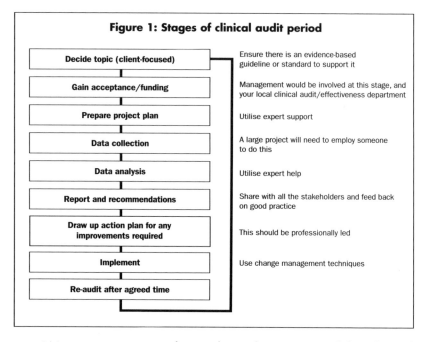

Figure 1: Stages of clinical audit period

Decide topic (client-focused)	Ensure there is an evidence-based guideline or standard to support it
Gain acceptance/funding	Management would be involved at this stage, and your local clinical audit/effectiveness department
Prepare project plan	Utilise expert support
Data collection	A large project will need to employ someone to do this
Data analysis	Utilise expert help
Report and recommendations	Share with all the stakeholders and feed back on good practice
Draw up action plan for any improvements required	This should be professionally led
Implement	Use change management techniques
Re-audit after agreed time	

We must now consider audit in the context of the clinical effectiveness process; as a method of evaluating the implementation of research evidence into practice. Sometimes, as in the case discussed in chapter 4 which concerned head lice management, base-line clinical audit is carried out to determine the current situation, or extent of need, before a standard is written. A future clinical audit can then audit the practice standard or guidelines and compare the change in practice against the first audit. An audit of current advised therapeutic interventions by community nurses for the management of head lice could be achieved cheaply and simply by using a questionnaire. The gains would be considerable in comparing the current situation against the recent evidence-based guidelines. A targeted programme of education, public and professional, could be instigated to overcome any discrepancies. The local management of head lice could then be re-audited.

In general when considering a clinical audit topic you need to ask the following questions.

- ○ Why is it important?
- ○ Does it affect a known quality issue?
- ○ Does it affect a large number of people?
- ○ Is it affected by variations in practice?
- ○ Is it a subject for local concern?
- ○ Will the gains, health and financial, justify the resources required to carry out the audit?

Before planning an audit it may be helpful to contact others who have performed similar audits. Some professional bodies hold a database of audits performed by their members.

Key success factors for audit[5,6]

- ○ Quality of leadership.*
- ○ Motivation and enthusiasm of staff.*
- ○ Support and commitment of senior management.
- ○ Active involvement of general management.
- ○ Publicised vision of objectives for audit.
- ○ Development of a questioning culture among staff.
- ○ Simultaneous consideration of professional, clinical, organisational and management aspects.
- ○ Prioritisation of issues and problems.
- ○ Realistic timescale and resources.
- ○ Awareness of ongoing process rather than one-off.
- ○ Suitably objective criteria/questions/standards with measurable components.
- ○ Measurement of the before situation.
- ○ Change targeted at the key deliverable.

* These will have the most impact on success.

Evaluation

A great deal has been written on evaluating health promotion and much of the methodology is relevant to community nursing practice. I want to introduce you to the model and types of evaluation as described by Anne Lazenbatt.[7] I believe that they offer a logical and necessary approach to the evaluation process for community nurses wanting to evaluate their services. The main aspects of evaluation she describes are needs assessment, structure, process and outcome evaluation. See Box 2 for definitions.

Evaluation can be short or long term. Long term outcome evaluation is particularly valuable as it demonstrates whether goals have been maintained over a long period of time. If you were evaluating an enuresis clinic not only would it be useful to know whether the child had achieved full bladder control after attending the clinic but it would be powerful evidence for continuing such a service if the bladder control was maintained over the next year. In this instance the evaluation would only involve a simple postal questionnaire one year after the last attendance.

The purpose of the evaluation will depend on what is being evaluated. You might be considering efficiency, effectiveness, value for money or equity of opportunity.[7] A good evaluation will use both qualitative and quantitative measurements; that is, it will examine facts and figures, and make an assessment of the views of the people involved with the intervention, both staff and their clients. From the results of the evaluation it is then possible to determine the strengths and weaknesses of the intervention. An action plan can be written to overcome the weaknesses and, as with clinical audit, the strengths should be fed back to those involved.

Evaluation should be built in at the start of any new initiative or practice change. This is particularly important for outcome evaluation which requires making a comparison. Involvement in evaluation is a powerful tool for learning and reflective practice. This is particularly so when public participation is sought. It is also a necessity for demonstrating the quality and value of community nursing services.

Box 2: Key aspects of evaluation[7]

Needs assessment

This discovers the baseline information against which the outcomes will be compared. It might consist of epidemiological data such as the current incidence of smoking among teenagers in the school to be targeted for a health education programme. Alternatively it could be a statement of the client's stated needs for health improvement. For example, the provision of a new local child health clinic.

Structured inputs

This includes the environment of the intervention and the resources required to plan and carry it out, staff equipment, building, skills. For example, an evaluation of child health clinics may involve looking at the suitability of the venue and the timing of the sessions.

Process

This is how the structured inputs are applied in order to achieve the intended outcomes. Every reader will be familiar with completing questionnaires following training. Such questionnaires usually examine the process of the training and sometimes also the structure. In the instance of the child health clinic process evaluation might examine the advice and information given by health visitors, general practitioners and practice nurses regarding weaning and nutrition.

Outcomes

These may be immediate, intermediate or long-term. Immediate and intermediate evaluation examines the early outcomes from the intervention such as an increase in knowledge regarding weaning or the number of clients attending the clinic who do not start their babies on solids before four months. Long-term evaluation might question whether parents were still following dietary advice given in clinic to prevent tooth decay two years later.

It is beyond the scope of this book to discuss evaluation methodology in depth but Figure 2 (over) illustrates the stages an evaluation could go through. A full evaluation will be time and resource-intensive so its potential value must be considered before it is undertaken. In the case of introducing a new service, setting up a pilot site and fully evaluating it could save resources in the longer term. A report of the whole systems approach to modernising health visiting and school nursing in Central Derby Primary Care Trust[8] makes interesting reading as it offers not only details of the change management process used and outcomes obtained but also chronicles the evaluation. Øvretveit[9] and Whitehead[10] offer other approaches to evaluation which are relevant to public health and community nursing evaluation.

Details of methodologies are available in textbooks of research methodology.[eg 11-13] As questionnaires are probably the commonest tool utilised for both audit and evaluation, the next section examines good questionnaire design.

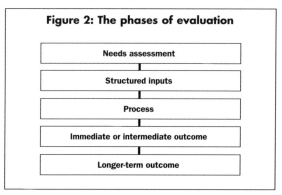

Figure 2: The phases of evaluation

Needs assessment

Structured inputs

Process

Immediate or intermediate outcome

Longer-term outcome

Designing questionaires

Good questionnaire design takes practice but will improve the value of the data you obtain immeasurably. A few important points to consider are:

- be sure of your objectives before writing the questionnaire
- consider whether to use open or closed questions. Open questions are good for exploring a topic but may be difficult or time-consuming to analyse. Closed questions are usually accompanied by alternative answers for the recipient to choose
- make your instructions and the layout clear
- questions must be explicit
- don't make the questionnaire too long
- always pilot your questionnaire with at least two or three people.

For further information see Oppenheim.[14]

Ethical approval

When planning any audit or evaluation you may need to consider whether you should seek ethical approval. When you are only using data that has been collected to care for the patient and the data collection is by the clinical team then this can be considered an extension of clinical practice. If, on the other hand, you decide to employ an external data collector to discuss aspects of their care with clients there may be serious ethical considerations. Client consent would be required and the client's general practitioner should be informed. The audit or evaluation plan should be referred to the local research and ethics committee. If in any doubt it is always worth contacting the ethics committee for advice. Further information on NHS systems for ethical approval can be accessed from the COREC website www.corec.com

Conclusion

Both audit and evaluation can be basic or detailed. If you are a novice start simply to build your confidence and try to work with a colleague or colleagues with some expert supervision.

Further information

Sources of support

Clinical audit/governance facilitators. Health care organisations have clinical governance departments with experts in clinical audit and evaluation methodologies. These staff are skilled in planning, carrying out and analysing the results of audits and will be able to guide and support you. In many instances it would be most appropriate to plan your audit in collaboration with the local clinical governance department.

Research and development departments. Many trusts have a research and development department. Most will be able to offer guidance on aspects of evaluation such as the choice of methodologies.

Universities Many trusts have a local university and close relations with it. Universities will be able to offer expertise in research methodologies.

Students A resource which might be exploited is the need of Masters and PhD students to complete a research dissertation. Many students struggle with finding a topic. It may be that a collaborative link could be made to a relevant university department and your evaluation might be taken on for such as dissertation. Almost certainly if you have a local university there will be local health professionals undertaking courses there. They might also be interested in your topic and could be contacted via a PCG/trust newsletter.

Clinical Audit Association Advice and training to support clinical audit. Tel: 01472 210682.

The Clinical Resource and Audit Group (CRAG). This is the lead body within the Scottish Executive Health Department promoting clinical effectiveness in Scotland. www.show.scot.nhs.uk/crag/main.htm.

Publications

Achieving Effective Practice: Parts 5 and 6. NHS Executive, 1998. Only available on the web: www.doh.gov.uk/pub/docs/doh.aep.pdf Straightforward guides written for nurses for designing and carrying out clinical audit and preparing an audit proposal.

Principles for Best Practice in Clinical Audit. National Institute for Clinical Excellence. Radcliffe, 2002. The latest text on clinical audit, written to provide a standard for best practice for all clinicians. It includes details of many helpful online resources to support the audit process.

Promoting Health: A Practical Guide. Ewles and Simnett. Scutari Press, 5th Edition 2002. A straightforward guide to evaluation of public health activities.

The Evaluation Handbook for Health Professionals. Anne Lazenbatt, Routledge 2002. A useful source of reference for those new to evaluation as well as more experienced managers and researchers.

Action Evaluation of Health Programmes and Changes. John Øvretveit 2002. Describes a user-focused action evaluation approach for evaluating health programmes, policies and changes.

References

1   NHS Executive. A first class service Leeds: NHS Executive, 1998.

2   NHS Executive. Clinical audit in the NHS. Using clinical audit in the NHS: a position statement. Leeds: NHS Executive, 1996.

3   Simnett I. Managing health promotion. Chichester: Wiley, 1995.

4   Dixon N. Good practice in clinical audit – a summary of selected literature to support criteria for clinical audit. London: National Centre for Clinical Audit, 1996.

5   NHS Management Executive. Framework of audit for nursing services. Leeds: NHS Management Executive, 1991.

6   National Institute for Clinical Excellence. Best Practice in Clinical Audit. Oxford: Radcliffe Medical Press, 2002.

7   Lazenbatt A. The Evaluation Handbook for Health Professionals. London: Routledge, 2002.

8   PHAAR Development Team. Modernising health visiting and school nursing practice. Central Derby Primary Care Trust 2003, www.southernderbyshire.nhs.uk

9   Øvretveit J. Action evaluation of health programmes and changes. Oxford: Radcliffe Medical Press, 2002.

10 Whitehead D. Evaluating health promotion: a model for nursing practice. *Journal of Advanced Nursing* 2003; 41.5: 490-498.

11 Abbott P, Sapsford R. Research methods for nurses and the caring professions. Buckingham: Open University Press, 2nd edition, 1998.

12 Robson C. Real World Research, Oxford: Blackwell, 2nd edition, 2002.

13 Carter Y, Thomas C (Ed) Research Methods in Primary Care. Oxford: Radcliffe Medical Press, 1997.

14 Oppenheim A. Questionnaire design and attitude measurement. London: Heinemann, 1966.

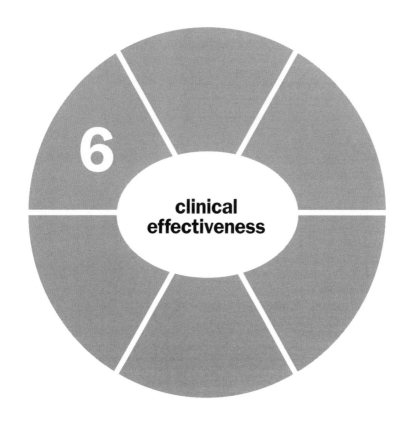

6

Disseminating successful outcomes

Just as important as questioning our own practice is sharing the outcomes with others. This chapter takes a practical look at the different techniques available for sharing outcomes. While successful outcomes should always be shared, it is useful to share failures as well as successes. In the past too much time has been spent reinventing the wheel or duplicating work. This is inevitable if we are unaware that the work has been done before. If the wheel is inefficient it may need reinventing but first its viability should be examined.

There are many reasons why our outcomes aren't shared, perhaps a major one being time constraints. Furthermore, it has often not been part of our working culture to prioritise the sharing of outcomes. The necessary skills are therefore not well developed. This must change. With the new agenda for health and nursing[1-3] clinical governance plays a pivotal role in improving health and reducing inequalities. Within the clinical governance agenda lifelong professional learning, sharing good practice and learning from experience are key objectives. Having learnt we must share that learning with others.

Before you read on...
In Table 1 is a list of some methods for disseminating outcomes. Consider, you are the person receiving information by these channels. Reflect on when this method of dissemination works for you and when it doesn't. Jot down your thoughts.

Table 1: Dissemination methods

○ one-to-one discussion
○ a report
○ a local presentation to your peer group
○ a conference paper
○ a journal article
○ a conference poster.

One-to-one discussion

Sharing your outcomes in discussion with another colleague is always worthwhile as it will bring another perspective and may alter your own interpretation. Indeed, this benefit is used in clinical supervision to improve practice. If you don't agree with one colleague's views, discuss your work with others and reach a consensus.

Chapter 1 discussed the benefits of forming a clinical effectiveness group to examine the evidence-base of professional practice. In this way a consensus is usually reached.

Once you have the confidence your outcomes are valued by local colleagues, consider how they could be disseminated to a wider audience. Remember negative outcomes can be as useful to learning as positive ones.

Sharing within your group

Professional time is always at a premium. For your colleagues to make time to hear about your work there must be an incentive for them to prioritise the time. Alternatively time can be prioritised for them if it becomes a management priority. Research on journal clubs[4] has highlighted that offering some form of refreshments for lunchtime meetings will improve attendance. Indeed, this is the approach adopted by many commercial companies. Would management sponsor a sandwich lunch? It's worth asking. Alternatively could you request a slot on the agenda of another regular meeting, generally well attended by your colleagues, for example, a staff meeting. Where the author worked in practice there were bi-monthly professional forums where projects could be presented and debated. Some branches provide a low-cost supper to attract attendance for evening meetings with speakers. This has the additional advantage of offering time for informal debate after the formal part of the meeting. The checklist for presentations is outlined in Table 2.

Table 2: Checklist for presentations

○ Prepare well in advance. You should spend 10 times as much time preparing as speaking.

○ Structure your presentation. Plan to tell the audience what you are going to say, say it, then tell them what you have said. That is, have an introduction, a main body and a conclusion (summary). It may be helpful to write down the main headings on cards which you can consult during the delivery.

○ Be sure of the main messages you want to get over, list them, then discuss them.

○ Prepare visual aids if they are appropriate. Make sure they are clear and not too wordy.

○ Practice, practice, practice. Time yourself and ask a friend to be the audience and give you feedback.

○ Think about what causes you most irritation when listening to other people's presentations and make sure you don't make the same mistakes.

○ Arrive in plenty of time to check the facilities and set up the room.

○ When delivering your presentation look at the audience and have eye contact with them. If you are very nervous look just above their heads!

○ Speak clearly and slowly. If ad libbing, be careful, it makes most presentations easier to listen to but can result in over-running the time available.

○ Try not to over-run, leaving time for questions.

○ Most audiences appreciate handouts.

○ Practice makes perfect so have a go.

Writing a local report

Submitting a report of your outcomes to senior managers, the Trust or health authority allows others, in this instance local policy makers, the opportunity to consider their value to local health care. The problem is that the readers will be extremely busy people who are likely to have a pile of reports on their desk.

Any report needs to be brief and clear. It should include a concise half page summary as many readers won't have time to read the whole report. In some instances it may be possible to summarise all your work on one or two pages. This will take you less time and it is more likely to be read. You can invite further contact if more details are required. Obviously a big project may require a full report but a brief one is preferable to no report if there are time constraints. Table 3 shows a standard report structure.

Table 3: A standard report structure is

○ summary of the project
○ introduction or rationale for undertaking the work
○ background reading, evidence base for the project
○ objectives
○ methodology
○ the results using diagrams as appropriate
○ discussion
○ recommendations including resource implications if possible
○ references.

When writing a report
○ be succinct
○ use headings and number paragraphs to keep points separate
○ emphasise your most important outcomes
○ don't draw conclusions from insufficient evidence.

Where possible organise a short local meeting (maximum one hour) to launch your report. Invite key stakeholders along (Box 1).

Box 1: Stakeholders

A stakeholder is someone who should have a personal or professional interest in your piece of work. It could be a consumer group, your manager, colleagues, a consultant, the director of public health, the PCT nurse representatives, your general manager, the executive nurse director, the PCT chair, patient representatives. If the project will need funding it is essential to include someone who can make funding decisions.

Further information on report writing can be found in the management section of most libraries.

Organising a stakeholders' meeting
Chose a convenient time and venue and plan well ahead to give those attending a chance to get it into their diaries. When you send out the invitations be clear why it will be worthwhile making the time to attend. Prepare your presentation carefully so that it is clear and to the point. It may be useful to use overheads. Present your findings and recommendations and invite questions. After the presentation those attending can be given copies of your report for further consideration. Copies can be sent to those sending apologies.

Writing for publication
This can seem very daunting but is a way of reaching a large audience. The biggest hurdles in getting started may be confidence and not knowing how to structure an article. Have a go – there are plenty of publications which can help.[5-7] Many journals will also help you if they feel the content of the paper will appeal to their readership.

The first step is to decide where you would like your paper to be published. This will depend on its academic status, the audience you want to target and the style of paper you want to write. Some journals publish in a much more informal style than others.

Discuss this with colleagues and visit the library to look at a range of journals. Having chosen the appropriate ones read the instructions for authors or if they aren't in that issue, ring the journal for a copy. Consider your material and decide which journal seems to most meet your objectives. If you are still unsure you can always ring or email the editor to see whether your article would be of interest.

You are now ready to write your article. Decide on which style is appropriate to your audience and the journal you are targeting. Then decide on the main message you want to convey and on the structure.

A formal research-based article should have a formal structure and style. Read some research articles to familiarise yourself with the format before starting if writing in this style. The standard format is:

- ○ synopsis
- ○ introduction
- ○ methodology
- ○ results
- ○ discussion
- ○ conclusion or recommendations.

It is very useful to make an article plan before writing. Having decided your main message you could put it in the centre of a spider diagram and decide what should be included in each paragraph as legs of the spider, for example. Alternatively, list the paragraphs. Different people develop their own styles.

You are then ready to start writing. Take your headings and write the paragraphs. Expect to have several drafts so don't spend too much time over the first one. It is more important to get the structure and flow organised. You can fine-tune the spelling and grammar later.

The most important aim of any article should be to make it appealing to the audience who will read it. This sounds logical but how often do you abandon interesting looking articles because they are too technical, wordy, full of jargon or lack anything new?

Once you have written the first draft I find that it is helpful to leave it at least overnight before beginning the process of fine-tuning. Once you are reasonably happy with your article ask a friend or colleague to read it, they will notice things which you haven't. Read it again yourself, in particular making sure that the meaning of each sentence is clear. Make final corrections and produce a final draft according to the instructions requested by the journal. Check the references carefully as poor referencing causes the biggest headaches for the editorial team.

Also don't forget to check spelling. I believe that

presentation is the key to success in this as in so many other areas of professional life. A well-presented, clear article must have more appeal than a poorly-presented one even if the content is the same. Use good quality paper, ensure that you have met the journal's criteria and attach a letter highlighting why you feel that this paper is relevant to the journal's audience.

If you would like further information or guidance why not do a 'Writing for Publication' course?

Submitting a conference poster

Over the past few years posters describing aspects of clinical practice have become a feature of many conferences. They have a number of advantages:

○ They provide an opportunity for face-to-face discussion of particular features of the project.
○ They are available for the whole conference so are more accessible to all those attending.
○ A large number can be accommodated while there will be restricted space on the programme for speakers.

There are disadvantages however:

○ The organisers may not value the posters as highly as the presented papers or the conference exhibition and they are consequently placed in a poor location.
○ The poster's authors will not be beside the poster throughout the conference and you may not manage to track them down.
○ Some posters are hard to interpret as they are too detailed and wordy.

It is important therefore that if you intend submitting a poster you are mindful of these issues. The first task is to get it accepted. Either respond to a call for posters which will be published in relevant journals, or if you are aware of a conference relevant to your topic contact the organisers and ask them if you can submit a poster. You will be asked to submit an abstract of your project which should include the project's objectives, brief background and details of the methodology, the outcomes and why they are important. This is usually limited to a maximum of 200 words.

If your poster is accepted then plan its content very carefully. The CPHVA has produced a fact sheet (no 4) to help www.amicus-cphva.org It should tell an interesting story. Consider the well-documented methods for getting health promotion messages across,[8,9] as these apply to any message. Diagrammatic representations of results are often quicker to understand than tables when time is at a premium. Consider the use of colour which will make it more attractive. If possible get it produced by an expert. To maximise its value include a contact name and address. Also state when you will be available to discuss its contents and prepare a one-page handout. There is nothing more disappointing than coming across an interesting poster and then discovering that there are no contact details for the authors. Worse still that there isn't even a handout so you can pursue its contents at a later date when you have more time. If these last points are adhered to then your poster will reach a much wider audience. Certainly I collect details of posters not relevant to me to pass on to other colleagues who may find them useful. I expect others do too.

Submitting a conference paper

The process for submitting a conference paper is similar to that for posters. Look out for a call for papers and then submit an abstract of your project to the organisers. Many conferences include concurrent sessions which are an opportunity for clinicians to present projects they have been involved with. These are often reasonably informal and should provide an opportunity for professional discussion. They are also a good place for your first presentation if you are nervous.

It may be that you feel that your work is worthy of a large audience and could form the basis of a keynote paper. Main papers should be especially inspiring and motivate the audience.

Table 4: Key points when preparing a conference abstract

○ keep it very brief

○ follow the instructions carefully

○ it must be word processed

○ use the title to demonstrate that the work is important, relevant, innovative and generalisable. It must catch the reviewer's eye

○ include the names of all those involved

○ keep a copy.

If you feel you could do this then discuss your ideas with the conference organisers. Usually, though, keynote speakers are invited speakers on specific topics relevant to the conference.

If you plan your presentation carefully and allow yourself plenty of time for practice there is no need to be nervous. Do check the audio-visual arrangements well in advance, however. There is nothing worse than arriving with overheads or a power point presentation only to find that there isn't a projector. When you arrive at the conference check again and find the person who will be responsible for the technical side of your session. Let them know what your requirements are in case special arrangements have to be made.

Remember to keep to your allotted time and try to engage the audience by eye contact and by what you say. Invite feedback either at the end of your delivery or after the session.

Who else is there?

We have discussed the usual dissemination channels but there are others to be considered. Professional bodies and the Department of Health are always interested in evaluated or innovative practice, particularly if it is presented in report form. National bodies need a perspective of what is going on in the field and will have their own means of disseminating your work. Your outcomes could influence policy decisions.

Professional bodies have close relations with the Department of Health. They are often approached to highlight examples of good practice to feed into government initiatives. They can only do this if they are aware of them. They are also approached by other bodies and journals wanting this type of information for projects they are undertaking. Let the information resources department of your professional body have a copy of your report. Make sure you include accurate contact details.

Use the media
The end point in practising clinically effectively is to improve the service we offer to our clients. If your team can demonstrate effective outcomes use the media to tell the public. Enlist the support of your public relations team and management to guide you. It raises staff morale and public confidence to read good news and it is good for the service.

General recap
However you decide to disseminate your outcomes, the following are useful points to inform your preparation:

- ◯ Decide on your main message and don't get distracted into lengthy discourse which will divert the audience from this message. Rather use opportunities to reinforce it.
- ◯ Know the needs of your audience.
- ◯ Think back to the exercise you undertook at the start of this book. What were the pitfalls? Avoid them. What made the method work for you? Build it in.
- ◯ Be systematic in your preparation.
- ◯ Be as brief as possible.
- ◯ Check clarity of your points with a colleague.
- ◯ Avoid jargon.
- ◯ Illustrate points with diagrams where possible.
- ◯ Keep it simple.

Good luck!

References

1   NHS Executive. The NHS Plan. The Stationery Office, 2000.

2   NHS Executive. A first class service. Leeds: NHS Executive, 1998.

3   Department of Health. Making a difference. London: The Stationery Office, 1999.

4   Bandolier 1997; 43.7. Oxford.

5   Cook R. The Writer's Manual. Oxford: Radcliffe Medical Press, 2000.

6   Hall G. How to write a paper London: BMJ Publishing, 2nd edition, 1998.

7   Albert T. Winning the publications game. Oxford: Radcliffe Medical Press, 1997.

8   Ewles L, Simnett I. Promoting health – a practical guide. London: Scutari Press, 5th edition, 2002.

9   Naidoo J, Wills J. Health promotion – foundations for practice. London: Bailliere Tindall, 2nd edition, 2000.

Index